Heartache to Healthy Heart
Cookbook:

Prevent, Reverse, and Fight Heart Disease With 30 Plant-Powered Breakfast Recipes.

NUEL VICTOR

Table of Contents

INTRODUCTION

For many people, breakfast is more than just food or the first meal of the day. It's a chance to give your body heart-healthy nutrients and start eating well all day. Consuming a nutritional breakfast that is based on plant-based foods will help to kickstart your metabolism, promote cardiovascular health, and give you with sustained energy throughout the morning.

This cookbook introduces a range of heart-healthy breakfast options and offers 30 delicious recipes, including energizing smoothies, overnight oats, and grain bowls, designed to keep your heart in top condition.

A heart-healthy breakfast focuses on incorporating whole, nutrient-dense foods that support cardiovascular health. These meals are rich in fiber, antioxidants, healthy fats, and plant-based proteins, which work together to lower cholesterol, reduce blood pressure, and minimize inflammation.

By starting your day with these nutrient-packed foods, you're not only nurturing your heart but also setting a healthful pattern for the rest of your day.

1. Berry Almond Overnight Oats

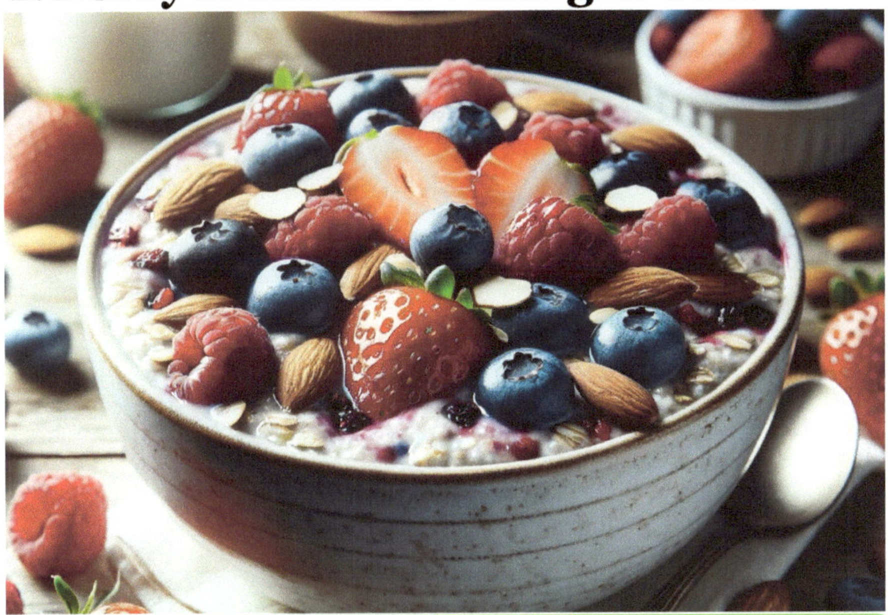

Ingredients

- Two tablespoons of sliced almonds
- Half a cup of mixed berries (either frozen or fresh),
- One tablespoon of maple syrup (if desired)

Prep Time: 5 Minutes

Preparation

- Combine oats, almond milk, chia seeds, and maple syrup in a jar.
- Refrigerate overnight. Top with berries and almonds before serving.

- Benefits:
Berry Almond Overnight Oats offer a significant heart health benefit primarily due to their high content of dietary fiber from both the oats and the berries. This dietary fiber helps to reduce cholesterol levels in the blood. Soluble fiber, found in oats, forms a gel-like substance in the digestive system. This gel-like substance binds to cholesterol and stops it from being absorbed, which makes it easier for the body to get rid of it. Getting less cholesterol makes it less likely that you will get heart disease, like coronary artery disease and stroke.

2. Green Smoothie Bowl

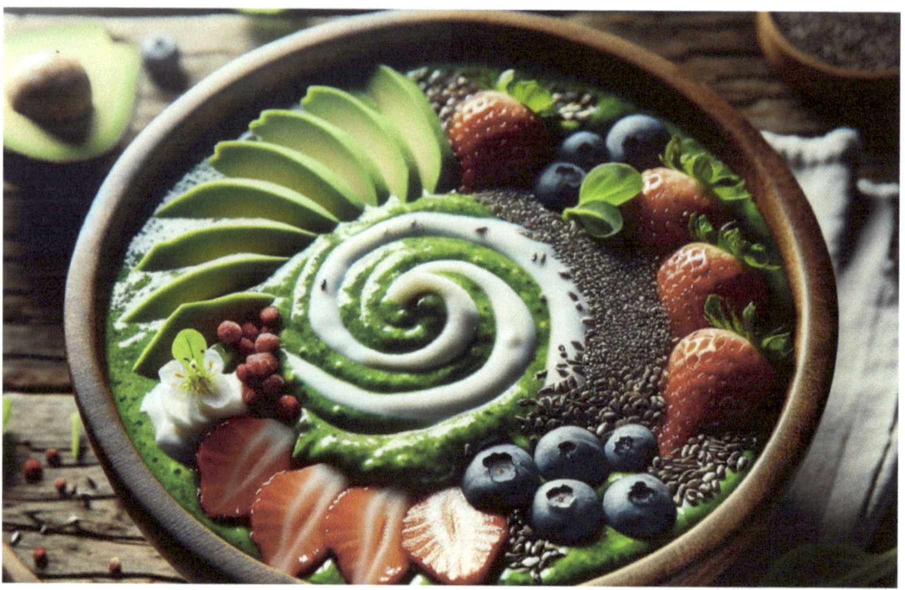

Ingredients

- 1 cup baby spinach,
- ½ ripe avocado,
- ½ banana,
- ½ cup unsweetened almond milk,
- ¼ cup frozen pineapple pieces,
- 1 tbsp flaxseed meal,
- Toppings: sliced kiwi, unsweetened coconut flakes, hemp seeds.

Preparation

- Blend spinach, avocado, banana, almond milk, pineapple, and flaxseed meal until smooth.
- Pour into a bowl and add toppings.

Prep Time:
Few Minutes

Benefits:
The Green Smoothie Bowl is rich in antioxidants and dietary fiber from its ingredients like spinach, kale, and fruits. Oxidative stress and inflammation, which cause heart disease, are reduced by antioxidants. However, dietary fiber lowers cholesterol, which prevents and reverses heart disease.

3. Chickpea Pancakes

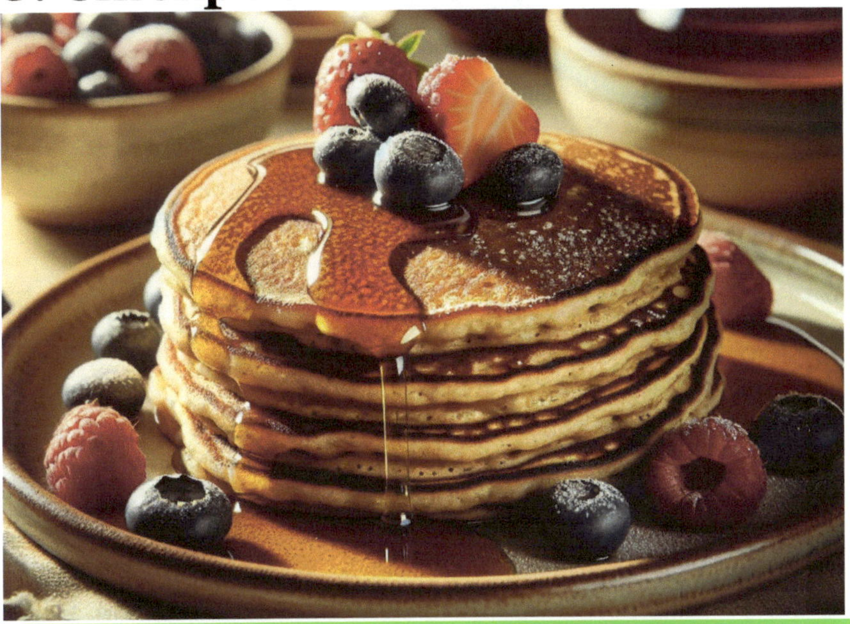

Ingredients

- Half a cup of mixed berries, which can be either frozen or fresh;
- two tablespoons of sliced almonds; and
- one tablespoon of maple syrup,
- If desired. Dice 1 cup of mixed veggies, like bell peppers, onions, and spinach.

Preparation

- Mix chickpea flour, water, nutritional yeast, turmeric, garlic powder, and salt.
- Cook pancakes on a non-stick skillet until golden on both sides.

Prep Time: 10 Minutes

Benefits:
Chickpea Pancakes are beneficial for preventing and reversing heart disease primarily due to their high content of soluble fiber. LDL cholesterol, which increases heart disease risk, is lowered by soluble fiber. When included in daily meals like pancakes, chickpeas' high fiber content improves heart health by lowering lipids.

4. Quinoa Breakfast Porridge

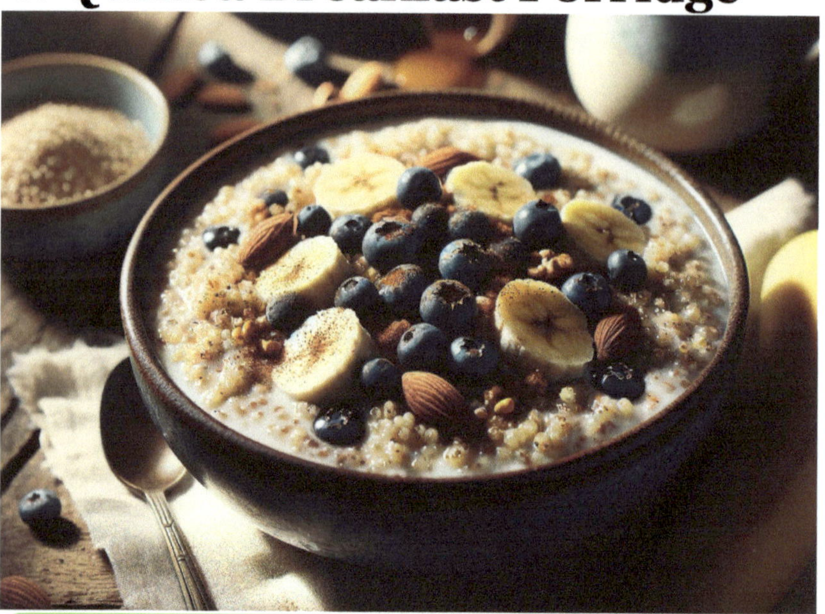

Ingredients

- ½ cup cooked quinoa,
- ¾ cup unsweetened soy milk,
- 1 tbsp almond butter,
- ½ apple, diced,
- 1 tbsp ground flaxseed,
- Cinnamon to taste.

Preparation

- Warm quinoa and soy milk.
- Stir in almond butter, apple, flaxseed, and cinnamon.

Prep Time: 10 Minutes

Benefits:
Quinoa Breakfast Porridge has a high content of anti-inflammatory phytonutrients, potentially beneficial for human health in the prevention and treatment of disease, and its small amounts of heart-healthy omega-3 fatty acids, along with a higher content of monounsaturated fat compared to common cereals, which can contribute to heart health

5. Avocado Toast with Tomato and Seeds

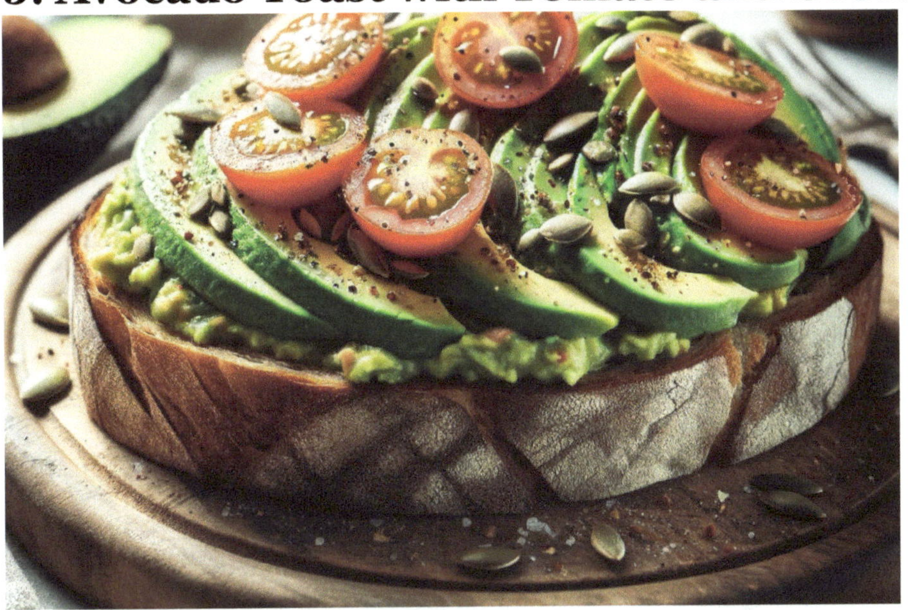

Ingredients

- 1 slice whole grain bread, toasted,
- ½ ripe avocado, mashed,
- ½ cup sliced cherry tomatoes,
- 1 tbsp pumpkin seeds,
- Salt and pepper to taste.

Preparation

- Spread mashed avocado on toast.
- Top with cherry tomatoes, pumpkin seeds, salt, and pepper.

Prep Time: 10 Minutes

Benefits:

- Avocado Toast contains monounsaturated fats like oleic acid, which reduce LDL cholesterol, a risk factor for coronary heart disease. To boost heart health and minimize cardiovascular disease risk, eat avocados, almonds, and seeds instead of saturated fats.

6. Tofu Scramble with Kale and Mushrooms

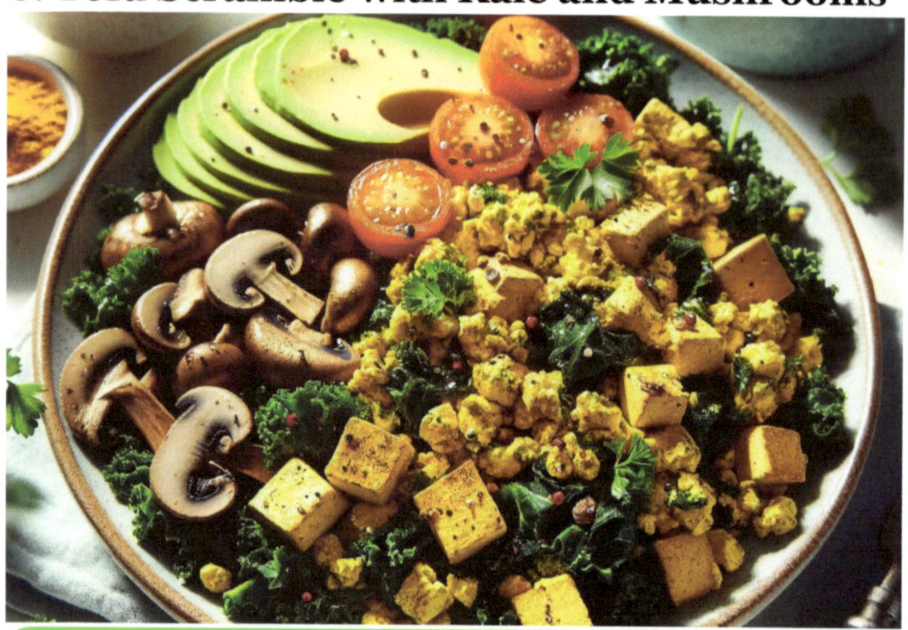

Ingredients

- ½ block firm tofu, crumbled,
- 1 cup chopped kale,
- ½ cup sliced mushrooms,
- ¼ onion, diced,
- 1 tsp turmeric,
- 1 tbsp nutritional yeast,
- Salt and pepper to taste.

Preparation

- Sauté onion, kale, and mushrooms.
- Add tofu, turmeric, nutritional yeast, salt, and pepper.
- Cook until heated through.

**Prep Time:
10 Minutes**

Benefits:

- Tofu, the main ingredient in Tofu Scramble with Kale and Mushrooms, helps prevent and treat heart disease. Soy plants produce estrogen-like isoflavones, which are found in tofu. Tofu may reduce heart disease risk in younger and postmenopausal women, according to research. Cardiovascular risk markers benefit from tofu isoflavones.

7. Chia and Berry Parfait

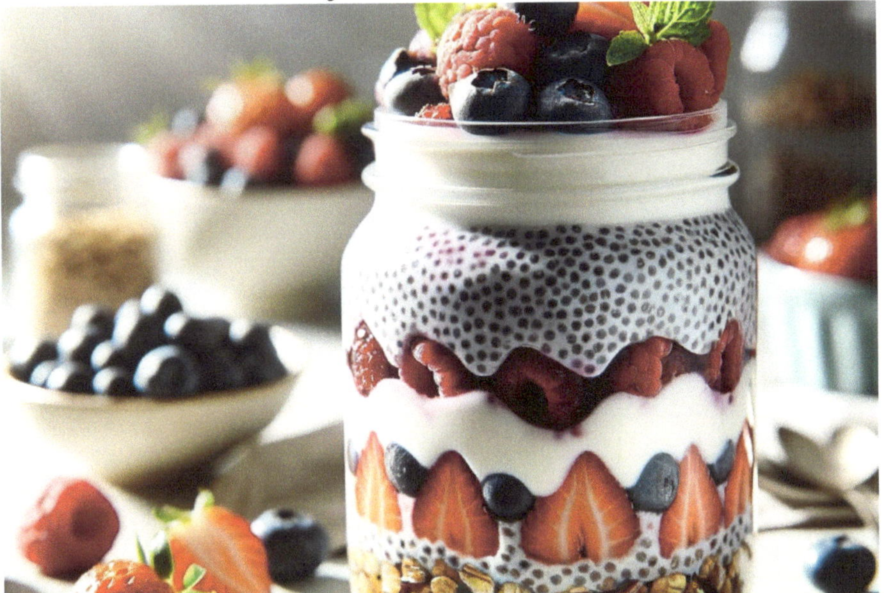

Ingredients

- 3/4 cup almond milk,
- 3/4 cup mixed berries,
- 1 tablespoon chopped almonds, and
- 1 teaspoon honey or maple syrup (optional).

Preparation

- Mix chia seeds with almond milk and let sit for an hour or overnight until gelatinous.
- Layer with berries and top with nuts and sweetener.

Prep Time: 10 Minutes

Benefits:

- Due to its heart-healthy elements, Chia and Berry Parfait can prevent and treat heart disease. Chia seeds contain omega-3 fatty acids, which reduce inflammation and improve heart health. Berries include antioxidants that decrease blood pressure and cholesterol, reducing heart disease risk.

8. Walnut Blueberry Oatmeal

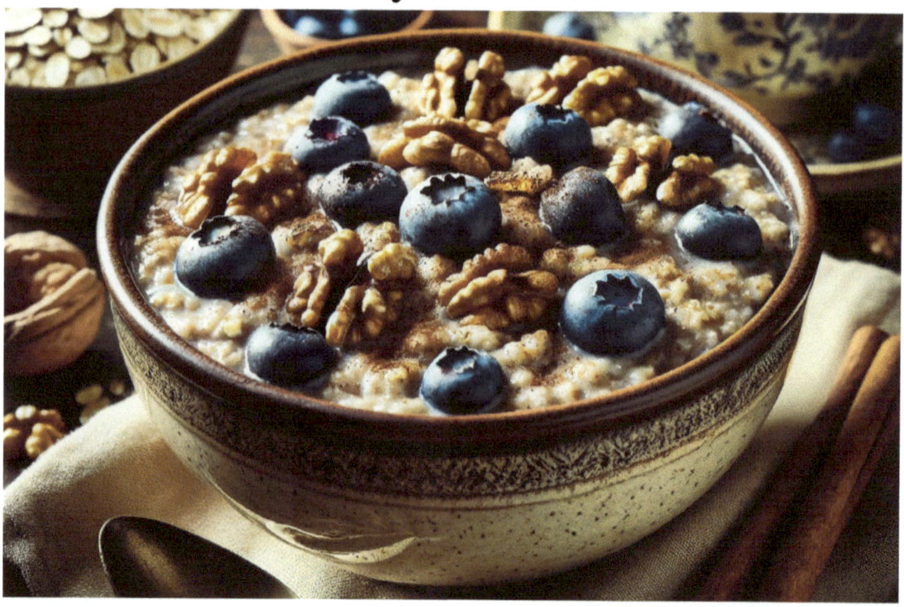

Ingredients

- ½ cup rolled oats,
- 1 cup water or unsweetened almond milk,
- ½ cup blueberries,
- 2 tbsp chopped walnuts,
- 1 tbsp ground flaxseed, Cinnamon to taste.

Preparation

- Cook oats with water or almond milk.
- Stir in blueberries, walnuts, flaxseed, and cinnamon.

Prep Time: 10 Minutes

Benefits:

- Walnut Blueberry Oatmeal can help prevent and reverse heart disease due to the combination of its key Ingredients. Beta-glucan, soluble fiber in oatmeal, lowers LDL ("bad") cholesterol and reduces heart disease risk. However, walnuts contain heart-healthy omega-3 fatty acids that cut LDL cholesterol and cardiovascular disease risk. Blueberries include antioxidants that reduce inflammation and enhance blood lipids, promoting heart health.

9. Sweet Potato and Black Bean Breakfast Burrito

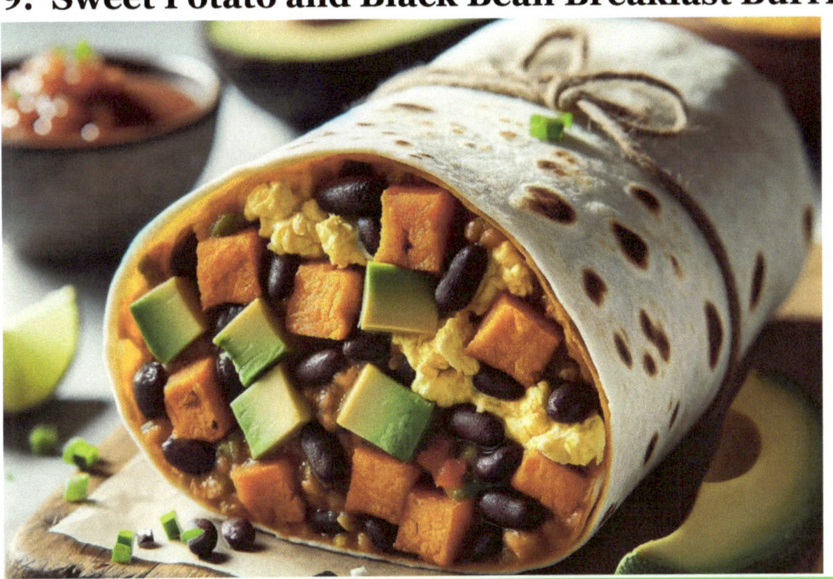

Ingredients

- 1 small sweet potato, diced and roasted,
- ½ cup black beans,
- 1 whole wheat tortilla,
- ¼ cup avocado, sliced,
- 2 tbsp salsa,
- 1 tbsp cilantro, chopped.

Preparation

- Warm tortilla.
- Fill with sweet potato, black beans, avocado, salsa, and cilantro.
- Roll up and serve.

**Prep Time:
10 Minutes**

Benefits:

Sweet Potato and Black Bean Breakfast Burrito can help prevent and reverse heart disease due to its nutritious ingredients. Sweet potatoes provide fiber, vitamins, and minerals, which lower heart disease risk. Black beans contain plant-based protein and fiber, which decrease cholesterol and enhance heart health. Spinach and avocado, which contain antioxidants and monounsaturated fats, also assist the heart.

10. Spinach and Mushroom Breakfast Muffins

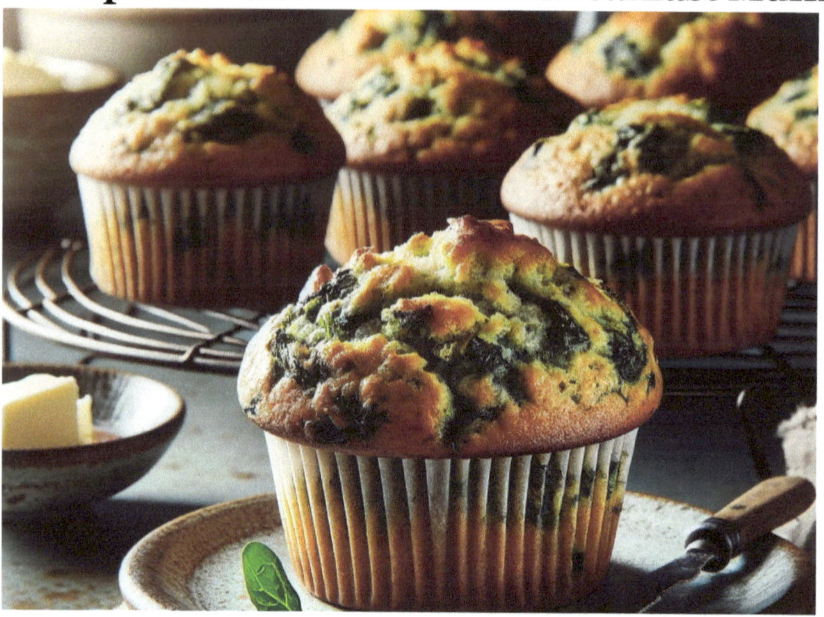

Ingredients

- 4 egg whites,
- 1 cup chopped spinach,
- ½ cup diced mushrooms,
- ¼ cup diced onions,
- Salt and pepper to taste.

Prep Time:
10 Minutes

Preparation

- Mix egg whites, spinach, mushrooms, and onions.
- Season with salt and pepper.
- Pour into muffin tins and bake at 350°F for 20 minutes.

Benefits:

- Spinach and Mushroom Breakfast Muffins can help prevent and reverse heart disease due to their nutritious ingredients. Mushrooms contain critical nutrients and lower heart disease risk, while spinach contains vitamins, minerals, and antioxidants. These muffins can also be part of a heart-healthy diet that includes whole grains and veggies, which lower heart disease risk.

11. Peanut Butter Banana Smoothie

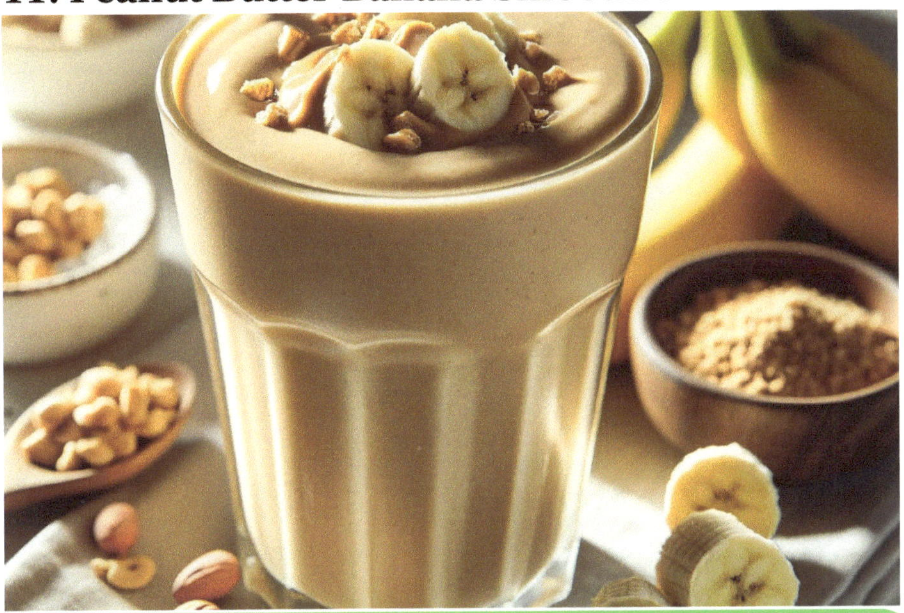

Ingredients

- A banana,
- A tablespoon of natural peanut butter,
- A cup of unsweetened almond milk,
- A tablespoon of ground flaxseed, and
- Ice cubes

Preparation

- Blend all ingredients until smooth.

Prep Time: 10 Minutes

Benefits:

- Peanut Butter Banana Smoothie can contribute to the prevention and reversal of heart disease due to its nutritious ingredients. Bananas contain potassium and fiber, which are excellent for the heart. Peanut butter provides protein, monounsaturated fats, vitamin E, and magnesium, which are good for the heart. Chia or flax seeds, with presence of omega-3 fatty acids and fiber, can also be added to the smoothie.

14

12. Mediterranean Veggie Hummus Toast

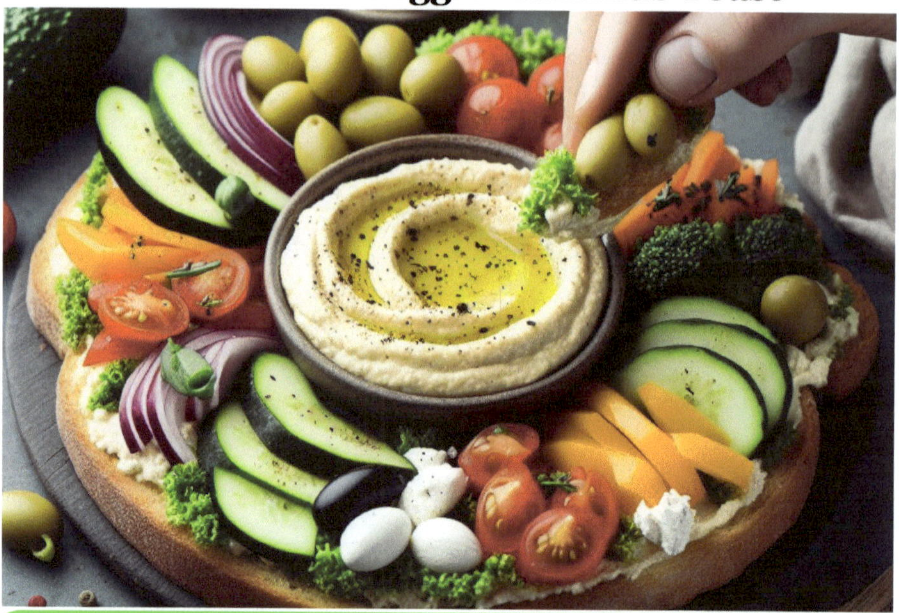

Ingredients

- 1 slice whole grain bread, toasted,
- 2 tbsp hummus,
- ¼ cup sliced cucumber,
- ¼ cup sliced tomatoes,
- 2 tbsp olives, chopped,
- 1 tbsp red onion, thinly sliced.

Preparation

- Spread hummus on toast. Top with cucumber, tomatoes, olives, and onion

Prep Time: 10 Minutes

Benefits:

- Mediterranean Veggie Hummus Toast can help prevent and reverse heart disease due to its nutritious ingredients and adherence to a Mediterranean-style diet. The Mediterranean diet, which is based on fruits, vegetables, whole grains, legumes, and healthy fats like olive oil, reduces heart disease risk. This dish uses chickpea hummus, which includes fiber and heart-healthy unsaturated fats. This toast also contains heart-healthy minerals and fiber from whole grains and vegetables.

15

13. Almond Butter and Jelly Oat Bars

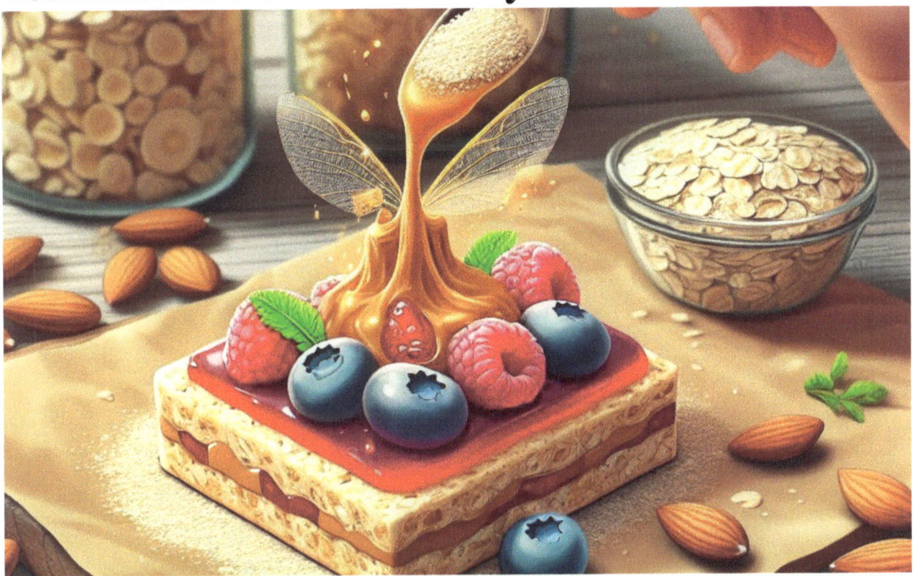

Ingredients

- 1 cup rolled oats,
- ½ cup almond butter,
- ¼ cup unsweetened apple sauce,
- 2 tbsp chia seeds,
- ¼ cup berry compote or low-sugar jelly.

Prep Time:
10 Minutes

Preparation

- Mix oats, almond butter, apple sauce, and chia seeds.
- Spread half in a pan, layer with compote, then top with remaining mixture.
- Bake at 350°F for 25 minutes.

Benefits:

- Almond Butter and Jelly Oat Bars' nutrients prevent and treat heart disease. Ground almond butter contains monounsaturated fats, omega-3 fatty acids, and vitamin E, which lower LDL and raise HDL. Oatmeal's fiber lowers cholesterol and prevents atherosclerosis. Additional heart-healthy components like berries and nuts can boost these bars' nutritional worth.

14. Savory Oatmeal with Avocado and Tomato

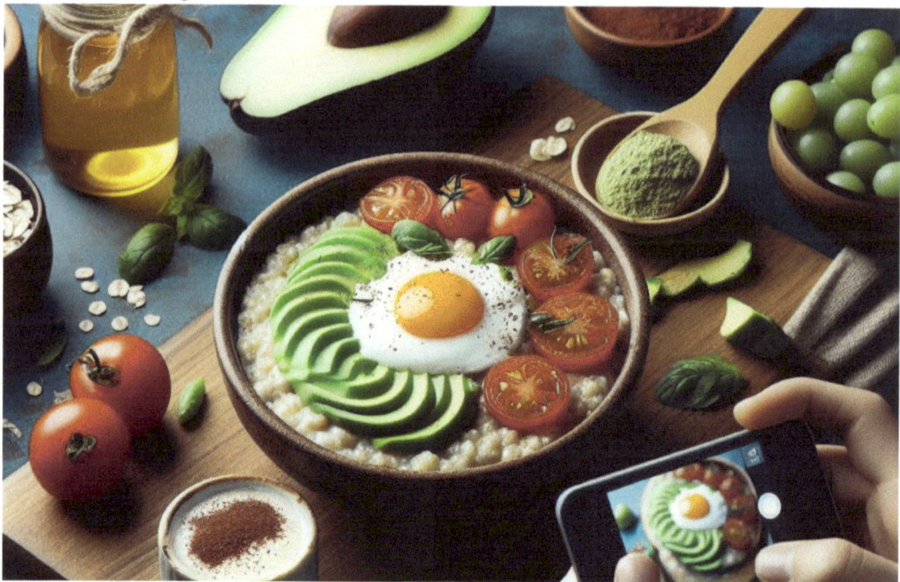

Ingredients

- ½ cup rolled oats,
- 1 cup water,
- Salt and pepper to taste,
- ½ avocado, sliced,
- ½ cup cherry tomatoes, halved,
- 1 tbsp pumpkin seeds.

Preparation

- Cook oats in water, seasoned with salt and pepper.
- Serve topped with avocado, tomatoes, and pumpkin seeds.

Prep Time: 10 Minutes

Benefits:

- Savory Oatmeal with Avocado and Tomato helps prevent and reverse heart disease thanks to its nutritional contents. Avocados include monounsaturated fats, which lessen heart disease risk and improve cardiovascular health. The carotenoid pigment in tomatoes, lycopene, may reduce inflammation helps to raise HDL cholesterol, and lessen heart disease risk. Oats, a healthy grain, also reduce LDL cholesterol and cleanse arteries, promoting heart health.

17

15. Berry Quinoa Salad

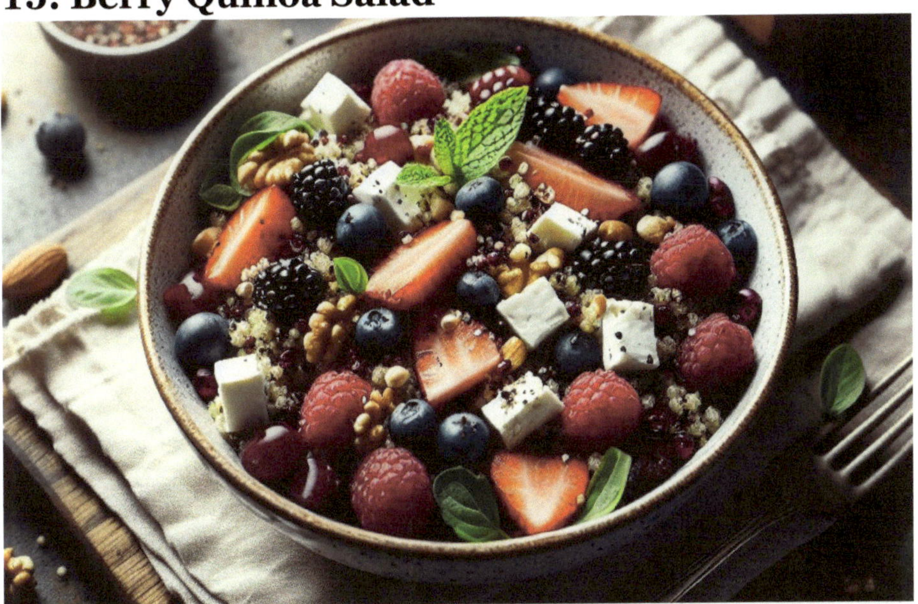

Ingredients

- ½ cup cooked quinoa, cooled,
- ½ cup mixed berries,
- 2 tbsp sliced almonds,
- 1 tbsp lemon juice,
- 1 tsp honey or maple syrup.

Preparation

- Mix quinoa, berries, and almonds.
- Dress with lemon juice and sweetener.

Prep Time: 10 Minutes

Benefits:

- Berry Due to its nutrients, quinoa salad can prevent and reverse heart disease. Antioxidants and vitamin C in blackberries and raspberries protect against heart disease and boosting heart health. Whole grains like quinoa provide fiber and plant-based protein, which are good for the heart. Heart-healthy components like leafy greens and citrus may boost the salad's nutrients.

16. Carrot Cake Smoothie

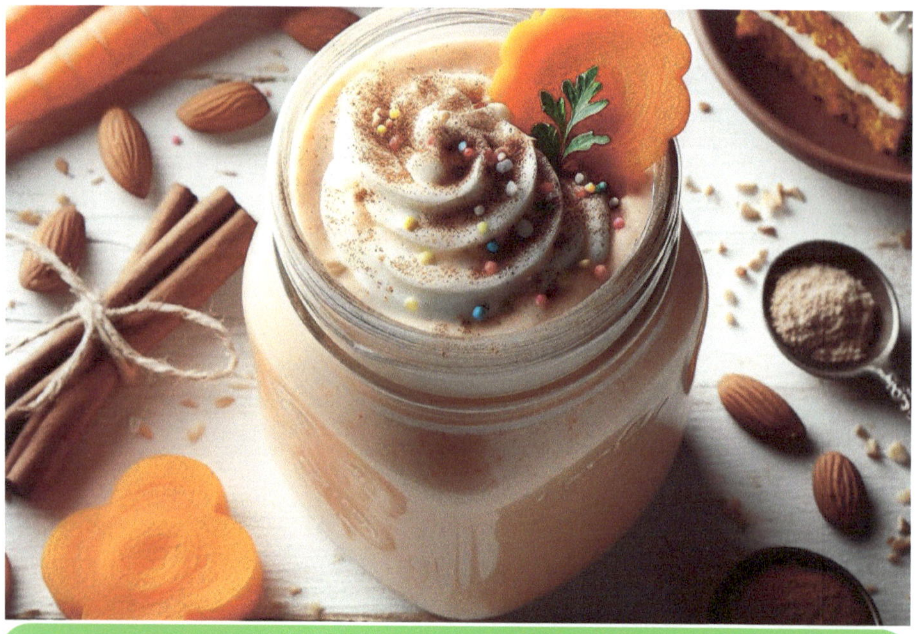

Ingredients

- 1 cup carrot juice,
- ½ banana,
- ¼ cup rolled oats,
- 2 tbsp walnuts, 1 tsp cinnamon,
- Ice cubes.

Preparation

- Blend all ingredients until smooth.

**Prep Time:
10 Minutes**

Benefits:
Due to its nutrients, Carrot Cake Smoothie can prevent and reverse heart disease. Beta-carotene, an antioxidant found in carrots, can reduce heart disease risk by avoiding oxidative damage and inflammation. Greek yogurt, which is high in protein and calcium, and walnuts, which are high in omega-3 fatty acids that reduce heart disease risk, may also be in the smoothie.

19

17. Zucchini Bread Oatmeal

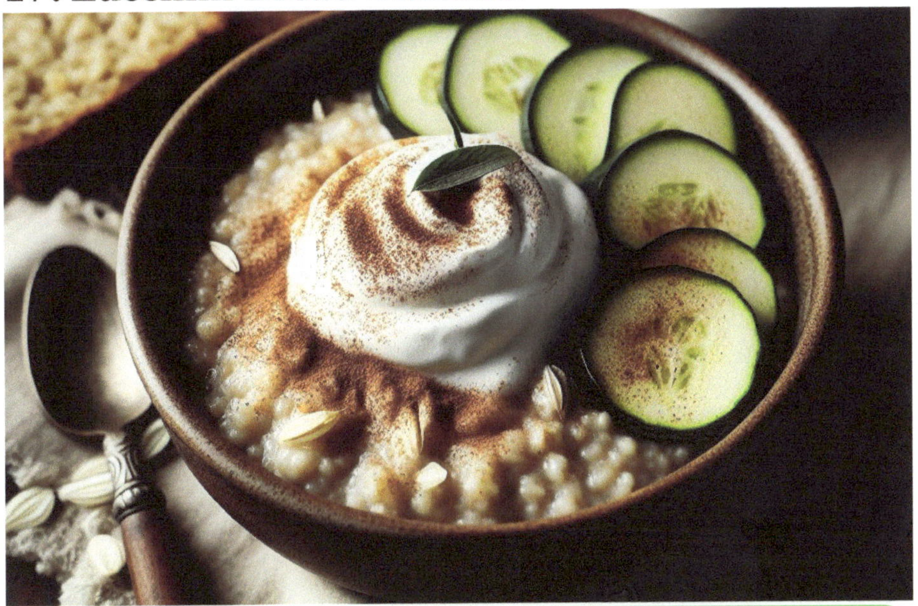

Ingredients

- ½ cup rolled oats,
- 1 cup water,
- ½ cup grated zucchini,
- 1 tsp cinnamon,
- 1 tbsp walnuts, chopped,
- 1 tsp honey or maple syrup.

Preparation

- Cook oats, water, zucchini, and cinnamon until oats are soft.
- Stir in walnuts and sweetener.

Prep Time:

10 Minutes

Benefits:

Zucchini Bread Due to its nutrients, oatmeal helps prevent and reverse heart disease. This recipe uses oatmeal, which is high in beta-glucan, a soluble fiber that lowers LDL cholesterol and heart disease risk. Zucchini adds moisture to oatmeal without adding a savory flavor, making it delightful and heart-healthy. This meal benefits cardiovascular health with fiber-rich oats and heart-protecting zucchini.

20

18. Vegan Breakfast Tacos

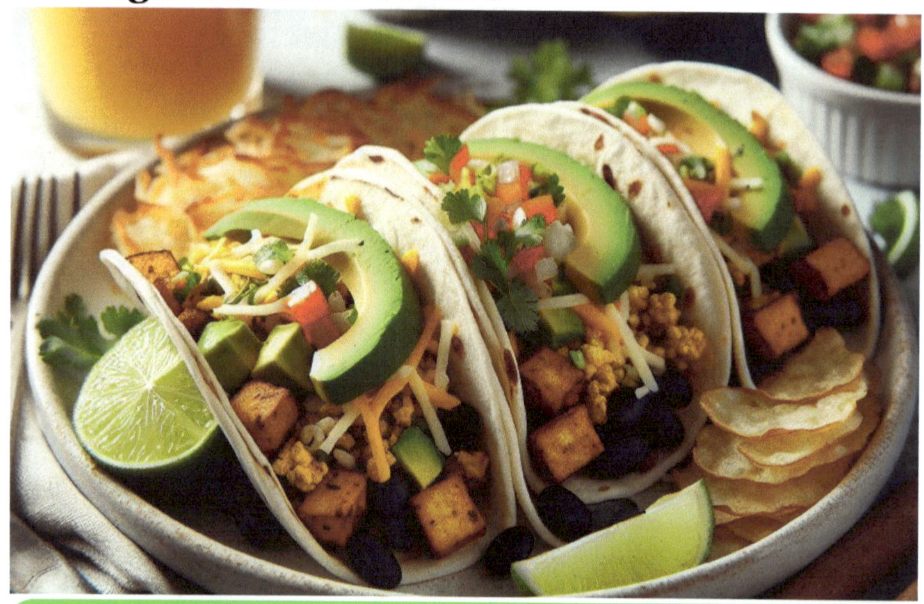

Ingredients

- 2 small corn tortillas,
- ½ cup tofu scramble,
- ¼ cup black beans,
- ¼ avocado, sliced,
- 2 tbsp salsa, Cilantro for garnish.

Preparation

- Fill tortillas with tofu scramble, black beans, avocado, and salsa.
- Garnish with cilantro.

Prep Time: 10 Minutes

Benefits:

- Vegan Breakfast Tacos' plant-based ingredients can prevent and reverse heart disease. Vegan diets improve cardiovascular health and reduce heart disease risk. Vegan breakfast tacos can deliver heart-healthy nutrients, fiber, and antioxidants by eliminating animal ingredients and adding veggies, lentils, and whole grains.

21

19. Pomegranate Pistachio Chia Pudding

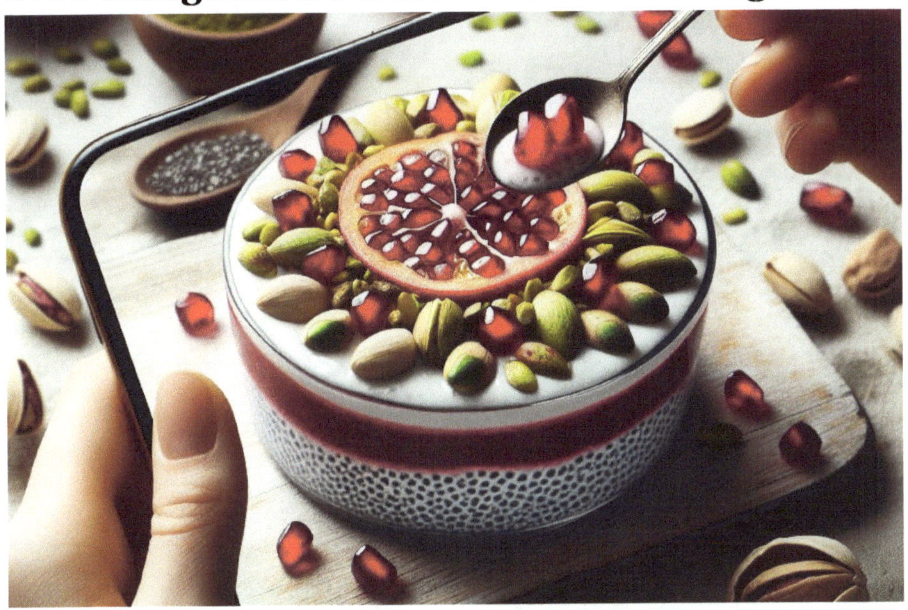

Ingredients

- 3 tbsp chia seeds,
- ¾ cup almond milk,
- ¼ cup pomegranate seeds,
- 2 tbsp pistachios, chopped,
- 1 tsp honey or maple syrup.

Preparation

- Mix chia seeds with almond milk and let sit to thicken.
- Top with pomegranate, pistachios, and sweetener.

Prep Time: 10 Minutes

Benefits:

- Due to its nutrients, Pomegranate Pistachio Chia Pudding may prevent and reverse heart disease. pomegranate antioxidants fight oxidative stress and inflammation, which can cause heart disease. Chia seeds also include fiber and omega-3 fatty acids, which boost heart health. The combination of heart-healthy components makes Pomegranate Pistachio Chia Pudding a good cardiovascular choice.

20. Mushroom and Spinach Breakfast Skillet

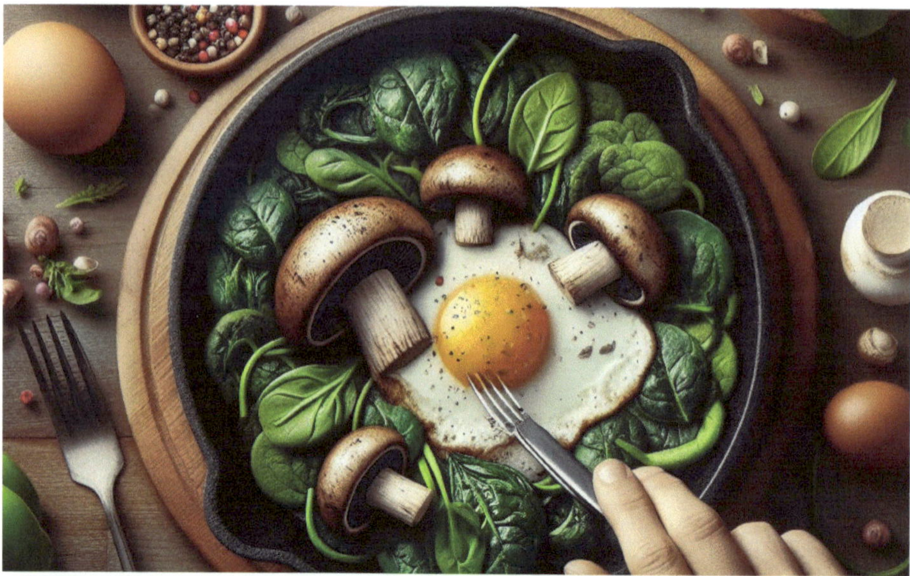

Ingredients

- 2 egg whites,
- 1/2 cup of diced potatoes,
- 1/4 cup of sliced mushrooms,
- 1/2 cup of spinach, salt and pepper to taste, and
- 1 tablespoon of olive oil.

Prep Time:

10 Minutes

Preparation

- Sauté potatoes and mushrooms in olive oil until tender.
- Add spinach and cook until wilted.
- Make wells, add egg whites, cover, and cook until set.

Benefits:

- Mushroom and Spinach Breakfast Skillet's healthy ingredients can prevent and reverse heart disease. Spinach contains heart-healthy vitamins and minerals like potassium and folate. However, mushrooms are low in calories and fat and contain antioxidants that prevent inflammation and oxidative stress, which are linked to heart disease. With these components, the morning skillet may be a heart-healthy portion of a balanced meal.

21. Apple Cinnamon Breakfast Quinoa

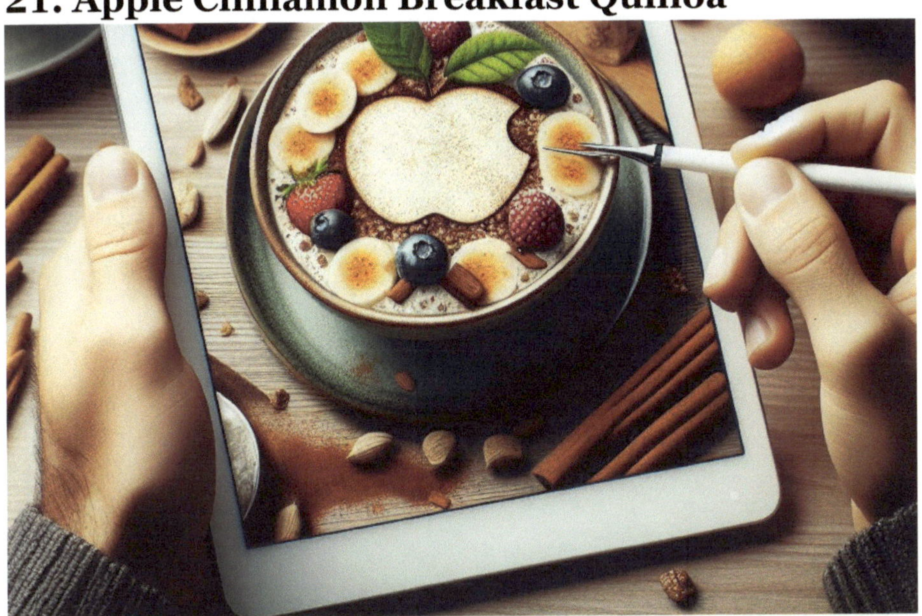

Ingredients

- ½ cup cooked quinoa,
- 1 apple, diced,
- 1 tsp cinnamon,
- 2 tbsp walnuts, chopped,
- ¾ cup unsweetened almond milk.

Preparation

- Warm quinoa with almond milk, apple, and cinnamon.
- Top with walnuts.

Prep Time: 10 Minutes

Benefits:

- Apple-Cinnamon Breakfast Due to its nutrients, quinoa can prevent and reverse heart disease. High in fiber and antioxidants, apples can lessen heart disease and other disease risk. Heart disease risk factors including cholesterol and triglycerides can be reduced with cinnamon, another essential component. Whole grains like quinoa are high in protein and fiber, which are good for the heart. By adding these heart-healthy elements to breakfast quinoa, it can improve cardiovascular health.

24

22. Veggie-Packed Breakfast Burrito

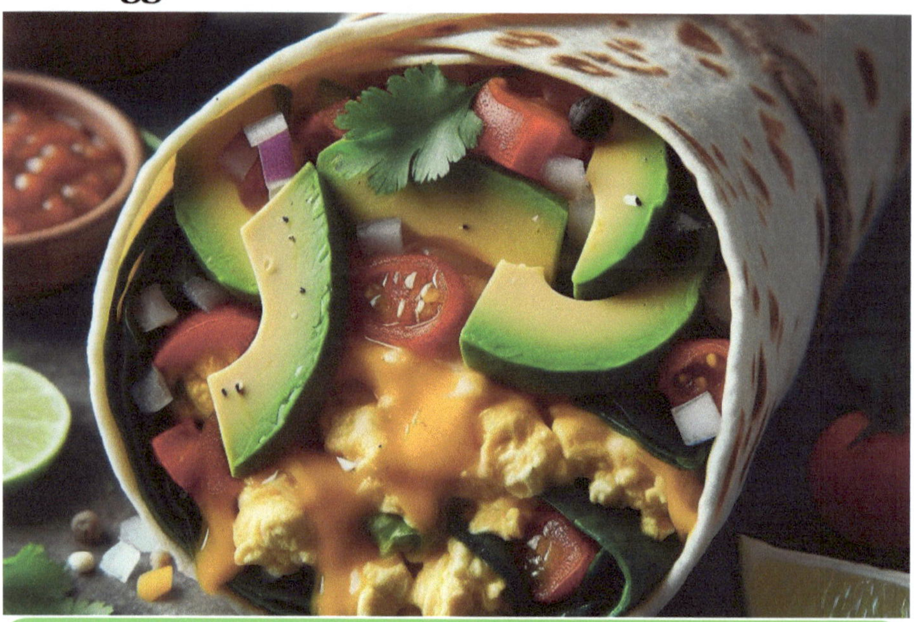

Ingredients

- 1 whole wheat tortilla,
- ½ cup scrambled egg whites,
- ¼ cup diced bell peppers,
- ¼ cup diced onions,
- ¼ cup spinach,
- 2 tbsp salsa.

Preparation

- Fill tortilla with egg whites, bell peppers, onions, spinach, and salsa.
- Roll up and serve.

Prep Time: 10 Minutes

Benefits:

- Veggie-Packed Breakfast Burrito's healthy elements can prevent and reverse heart disease. Bell peppers, spinach, and tomatoes deliver heart-healthy vitamins, minerals, and antioxidants. By replacing animal-based proteins with tofu or beans, this tortilla can cut cholesterol and saturated fat, lowering heart disease risk. This breakfast burrito is good for your heart since it has fiber-rich vegetables and plant-based proteins.

23. Raspberry Almond Chia Smoothie

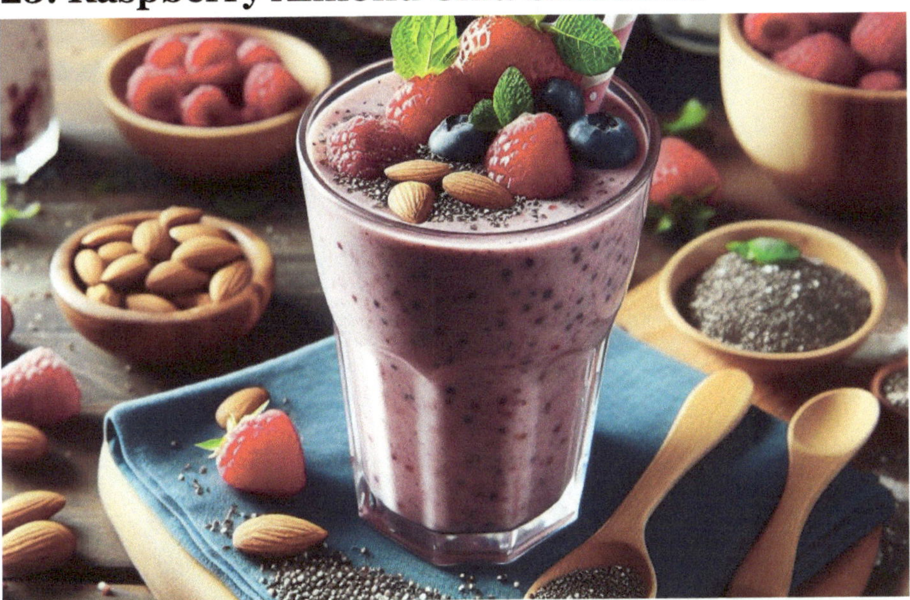

Ingredients

- 1 cup unsweetened almond milk,
- ½ cup raspberries,
- 1 banana,
- 2 tbsp chia seeds,
- 1 tbsp almond butter,
- Ice cubes.

Preparation

- Blend all ingredients until smooth.

Prep Time: 5 Minutes

Benefits:

Due to its nutrients, Raspberry Almond Chia Smoothie may prevent and reverse heart disease. Chia seeds in this smoothie are high in fiber and antioxidants and can improve insulin resistance, blood sugar, and inflammation, which are linked to heart disease. Almonds provide protein and healthy fats, while raspberries deliver antioxidants and fiber for heart health. Adding these heart-healthy elements to the smoothie can improve cardiovascular health.

26

24. Pear and Walnut Toast

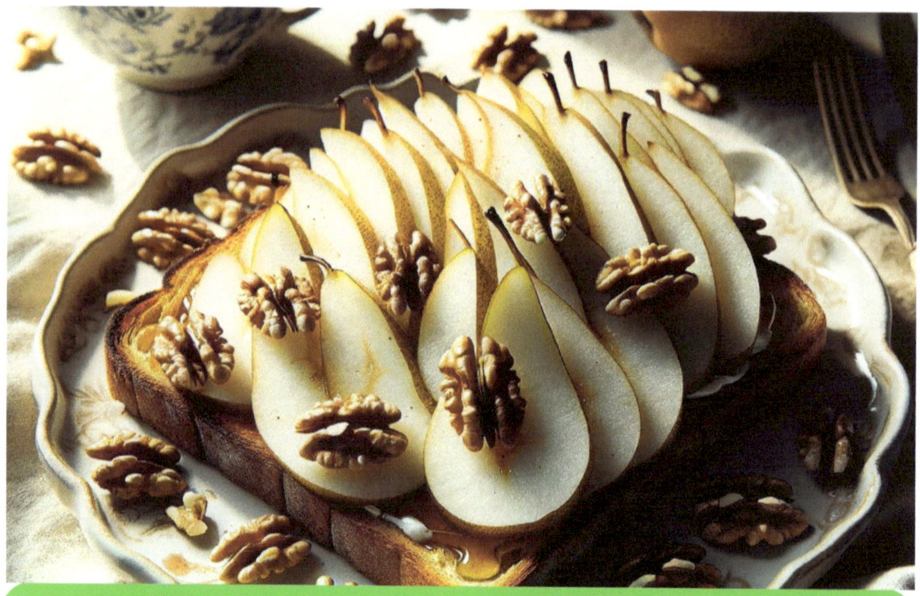

Ingredients

- 1 slice whole grain bread, toasted,
- 1 pear, thinly sliced,
- 2 tbsp ricotta cheese,
- 2 tbsp walnuts, chopped,
- Honey drizzle (optional).

Preparation

- Spread ricotta on toast.
- Top with pear slices, walnuts, and honey.

Prep Time:

7 Minutes

Benefits:

- Walnut, Pear Toast can prevent and reverse heart disease because of its nutrients. This toast contains walnuts, which include unsaturated fats like omega-3 fatty acids, which can lower LDL cholesterol, raise HDL cholesterol, and prevent irregular heart beats. Pears include fiber and heart-healthy minerals. Adding these heart-healthy items to toast can improve cardiovascular health.

27

25. Spinach and White Bean Breakfast Hash

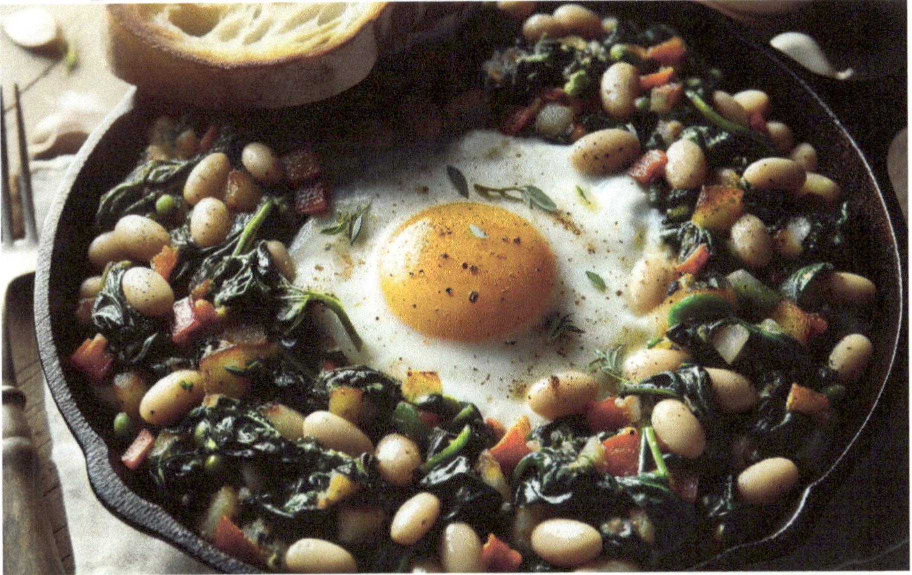

Ingredients

- ½ cup canned white beans, rinsed,
- 1 cup spinach,
- ½ cup diced sweet potatoes, roasted,
- 1 tbsp olive oil,
- Salt and pepper to taste.

Prep Time:
7 Minutes

Preparation

- Sauté sweet potatoes and white beans in olive oil.
- Add spinach and cook until wilted.
- Season with salt and pepper.

Benefits:

- Due to its nutrients, Spinach and White Bean Breakfast Hash helps prevent and reverse heart disease. Spinach has vitamins, minerals, and antioxidants, while white beans lower cholesterol with fiber and plant-based protein. Heart disease risk is reduced by eating a plant-based breakfast like this hash with nutritious grains and vegetables.

26. Blueberry Flax Microwave Muffin

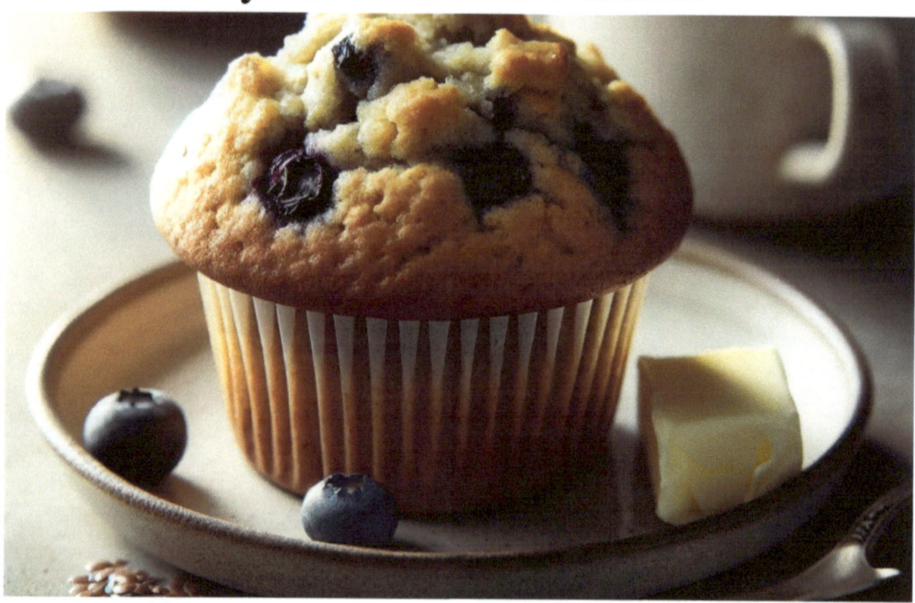

Ingredients

- ¼ cup ground flaxseed,
- 1 egg white,
- ½ banana, mashed,
- ½ tsp baking powder,
- ¼ cup blueberries,
- 1 tsp honey or maple syrup.

Preparation

- Mix flaxseed, egg white, banana, and baking powder in a mug.
- Fold in blueberries.
- Microwave on high for 2-3 minutes.

Prep Time: 7 Minutes

Benefits:

- Blueberry Flax Microwave Muffin can contribute to the prevention and reversal of heart disease due to its nutritious ingredients. This muffin contains flaxseed, which contains omega-3 fatty acids and fiber, which lower blood pressure, inflammation, and heart health. Additionally, blueberries are packed with antioxidants that have been shown to support cardiovascular health. By incorporating these heart-healthy ingredients into the muffin, it can be a beneficial choice for cardiovascular well-being.

29

27. Cucumber Avocado Toast

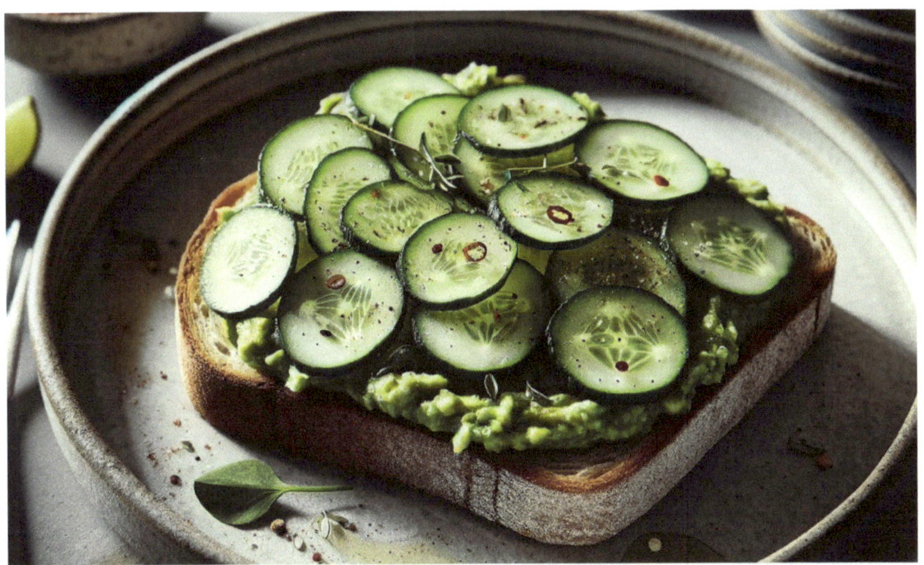

Ingredients

- 1 slice whole grain bread, toasted,
- ½ avocado, mashed,
- ¼ cucumber, sliced,
- Salt and pepper to taste,
- Red pepper flakes (optional).

Preparation

- Spread mashed avocado on toast.
- Top with cucumber slices, salt, pepper, and red pepper flakes.

Prep Time: 7 Minutes

Benefits:

- Cucumber Avocado Toast can contribute to the prevention and reversal of heart disease due to its nutritious ingredients. Avocado, a significant ingredient in this toast, has monounsaturated fats that boost heart health and lessen cardiovascular disease risk. Cucumbers are hydrating and rich in vitamins and minerals that assist cardiovascular health. By adding these heart-healthy elements to toast, it can improve heart health.

30

28. Vegan Protein-Packed Smoothie Bowl

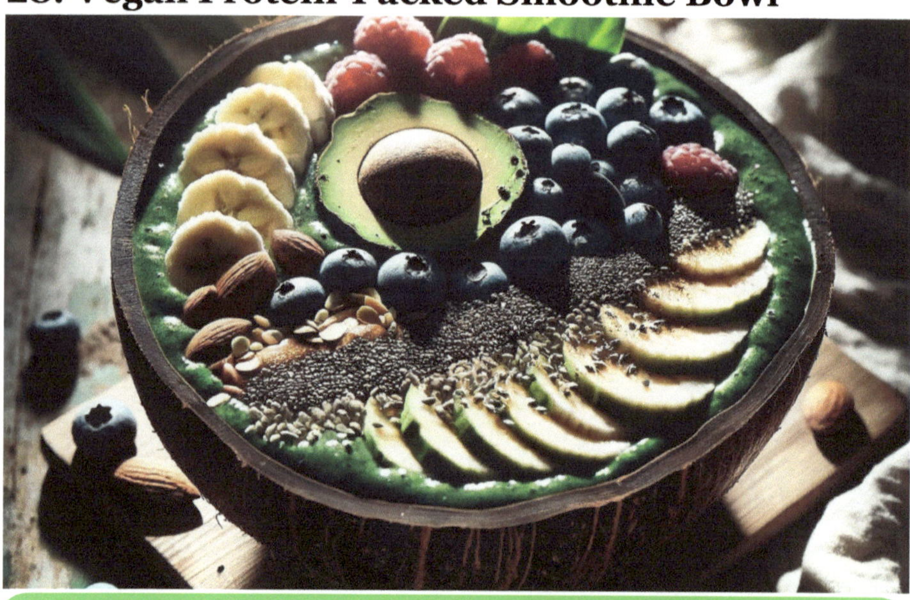

Ingredients

- 1 cup unsweetened soy milk,
- 1 frozen banana,
- ½ cup frozen mixed berries,
- 1 scoop plant-based protein powder,
- Toppings: granola, sliced almonds, hemp seeds.

Preparation

- Blend soy milk, banana, berries, and protein powder until smooth.
- Pour into a bowl and add toppings.

Prep Time: 3 Minutes

Benefits:

- A Vegan Protein-Packed Smoothie Bowl can contribute to the prevention and reversal of heart disease due to its nutritious ingredients. Vegan diets reduce heart disease risk and promote cardiovascular health. Minerals, fiber, and antioxidants that are good for the heart are found in fruits, vegetables, whole grains, legumes, and nuts. Including a vegan protein-packed smoothie bowl in your diet can boost your heart health.

29. Tomato Basil Omelet (Egg Whites)

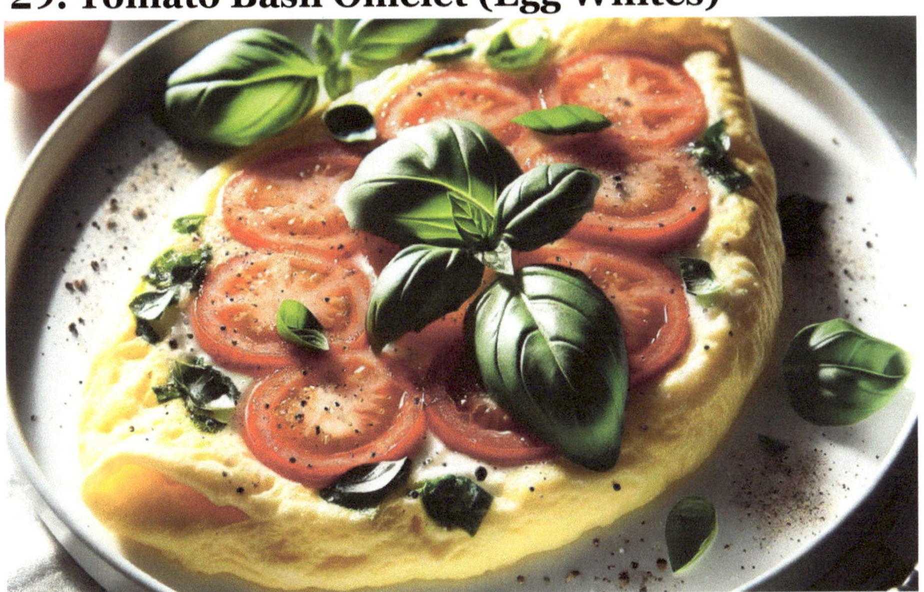

Ingredients

- Three egg whites,
- half a cup of diced tomatoes,
- two tablespoons of chopped fresh basil,
- salt and pepper to taste,
- and one teaspoon of olive oil.

Preparation

- Whisk egg whites with salt and pepper.
- Cook in olive oil, adding tomatoes and basil before folding.

Prep Time: 5 Minutes

Benefits:

- A Tomato Basil Omelet cooked with egg whites helps prevent and reverse heart disease thanks to its nutritional contents. Egg whites are low in cholesterol and saturated fat, heart disease risk factors. Additionally, tomatoes and basil provide antioxidants and other beneficial compounds that support cardiovascular health By incorporating these heart-healthy ingredients into the omelet, it can be a nutritious choice for heart health.

30. Kiwi Spinach Smoothie

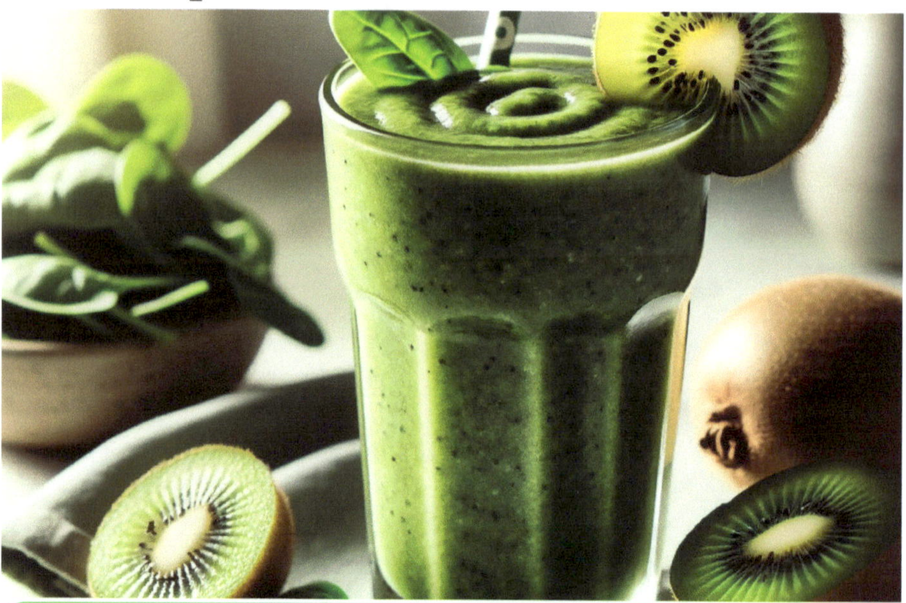

Ingredients

- 1 cup fresh spinach,
- 2 kiwis, peeled and sliced,
- ½ banana,
- 1 cup unsweetened almond milk,
- 1 tbsp ground flaxseed,
- Ice cubes.

Preparation

- Blend all ingredients until smooth.

**Prep Time:
7 Minutes**

Benefits:

- A Kiwi Spinach Smoothie can contribute to the prevention and reversal of heart disease due to its nutritious ingredients. Kiwis has a high presence of vitamin C, fiber, and antioxidants, which boost cardiovascular health and reduce heart disease risk. Spinach, on the other hand, is rich in heart-healthy vitamins, minerals, and antioxidants. By incorporating these heart-healthy ingredients into the smoothie, it can be a beneficial choice for cardiovascular well-being.

Final Thougts

These recipes are designed to provide a heart-healthy start to your day, incorporating ingredients that support cardiovascular health. Enjoy these meals as you embark on a journey to better heart health through nutrition.

Your cardiovascular health can be supported from the beginning of the day by incorporating heart-healthy foods into your breakfast routine. This is a straightforward yet effective strategy to support your cardiovascular health.

These 30 recipes offer a variety of flavors and nutrients designed to cater to different tastes and preferences while focusing on heart health. You can enjoy tasty and gratifying meals that not only taste good but also do good for your heart if you use ingredients that are derived from plants and are rich in nutrients.